Oumaima Tayari
Amel Hamza

Which supra-implant prosthesis should be indicated for a fully edentulous patient?

Oumaima Tayari
Amel Hamza

Which supra-implant prosthesis should be indicated for a fully edentulous patient?

ScienciaScripts

Publisher:
Sciencia Scripts
is a trademark of
Dodo Books Indian Ocean Ltd. and OmniScriptum S.R.L publishing group

120 High Road, East Finchley, London, N2 9ED, United Kingdom
Str. Armeneasca 28/1, office 1, Chisinau MD-2012, Republic of Moldova, Europe
Printed at: see last page
ISBN: 978-620-3-69545-8

CONTENTS

INTRODUCTION

According to the criteria of the World Health Organisation (WHO), a completely edentulous patient is considered to be physically deficient and disabled, and complete edentulism constitutes a functional handicap, social and psychological problems. In order to improve the quality of life of these patients, oral rehabilitation is necessary(22) (38). Progress in the field of oral rehabilitation of the edentulous was initiated more than 50 years ago. Thanks to implantology, edentulous patients can benefit from improved oral care. Brånemark, the pioneer of modern implant dentistry, used titanium implants mainly in edentulous arches. Clinical results up to 15 years follow-up were very promising, particularly in the edentulous mandible (11). Similarly, there are now various prosthetic-implant solutions available to dentists for rehabilitating the completely edentulous arch, especially as the results of several randomised studies with short- and long-term follow-up have confirmed that implant-supported prostheses are more beneficial than conventional prostheses. (20)These prostheses offer functional and biological advantages over conventional prostheses, such as a reduction in the rate of bone resorption, improved retention and stability, improved masticatory efficiency, and a reduction in soft tissue trauma, all of which considerably improve the quality of life of many patients. (20) (63) The success of a total supra-implant prosthesis depends essentially on the validation of the choice of the type of prosthesis to be indicated, which justifies the importance of the preoperative phase in identifying the various factors influencing the prosthetic decision, the treatment plan and the operative follow-up. In this study, we will attempt to describe the possible supra-implant prosthetic alternatives for complete prostheses. Then, we will determine the decision-making criteria for these prosthetic choices. Finally, we will detail the most important points in the preoperative assessment of any edentulous patient undergoing prosthetic-implant rehabilitation.

CHAPTER 1

THE DIFFERENT TYPES OF SUPRA-IMPLANT PROSTHESES IN THE EDENTULOUS PATIENT

Implantology offers several prosthetic solutions for the rehabilitation of edentulous teeth. These can be fixed, removable or non-removable.

1-1- Removable solution

1-1-1- Complete removable supra-implant prosthesis (PACSI) with additional retention :

The retention and stability of conventional complete prostheses pose a major challenge. more problems in the mandible than in the maxilla. This is mainly due to the reduced bearing surface in the mandibular arch. As a result, implant-supported prostheses are a more reliable treatment for edentulous arches. Indeed, the 2002 McGill Consensus Conference concluded that mandibular PACSI supported by two symphyseal implants is considered the minimum acceptable treatment to compensate for mandibular edentulism and offers excellent long-term survival rates. (58) (13,59)
The PACSI is a conventional complete removable prosthesis that covers implants which act as a retention complement.(61) In fact, with the PACSI, in order to respond to the principle of Housset's triad: support and stabilisation are provided by the osteofibromucosal tissues while retention is enhanced by an attachment system connected to the implants. (21) The degree of retention depends on the design, position and alignment of the implants and the type of attachment system chosen(53) (54). Implants can be :

*are disconnected: this is the case with unitary systems based on the "snap-fit" principle with axial attachments.
*are connected by a bar that holds them together(10).

❖ Axial attachments: Definition :

These attachments are mechanical connections comprising a patrix (part) that fits into a matrix (female part). The male part is generally included in the prosthetic base either by indirect technique in the laboratory or by direct technique in the chair. Retention is obtained by interlocking the male and female parts.(1) (21) Several types of axial attachment are available. They differ in the

3

method of retention:

■Direct friction force between the male and female parts obtained by
activatable metal strips (DALBO B®) or non-activatable plastic ties (retention sheaths). (LOCATOR®)

■Locking between a female part consisting of a housing comprising
a silicone ring and a spherical male part (O'RING®)

■Magnet systems: Retention is ensured by a magnetic field. These systems have been abandoned. (1)

Ball attachment:

This is a resilient axial attachment allowing vertical translation and distal rotation. It consists of a female part comprising a housing with a synthetic ring and a male part formed by a spherical abutment screwed onto the implant. Retention is achieved by locking these two parts together. The rings are perceived as being consumable, as they will be replaced as soon as signs of wear and loss of retention become apparent. (66) (57). **(Fig.1)**

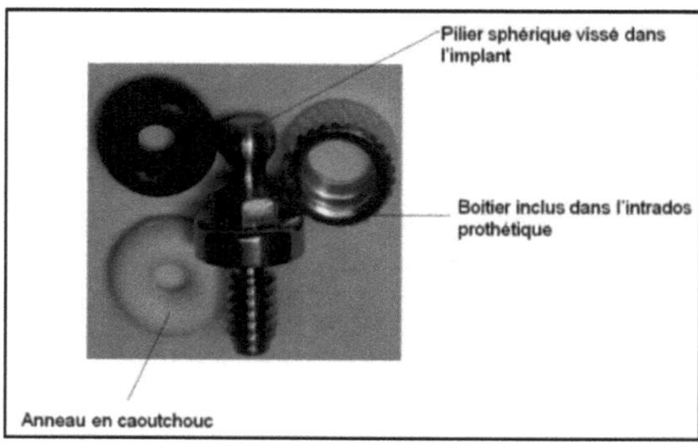

Figure 1: Example of the components of a ball attachment (O'RING)(57)

LOCATOR attachment:

This is a resilient cylindrical axial attachment. It is made up of a Locator abutment (matrix) fixed at the implant connection and a titanium case included in the prosthetic intrados where retention sleeves (patrice) are inserted. (fig. 2) These retention sleeves are nylon inserts with different retention strengths, marked by different colours and chosen according to the angulation of the implants. (1) This type of attachment was used in the first case described above. The EQUATOR ASTRA ACQUA ® brand attachment system allows correction of up to 35° of divergence between two implants and has 4 retention sheaths adapted to different clinical situations: the yellow sheath (with the least retention) was chosen to allow easy insertion and removal for the patient given that she lacks manual dexterity due to Parkinson's disease.

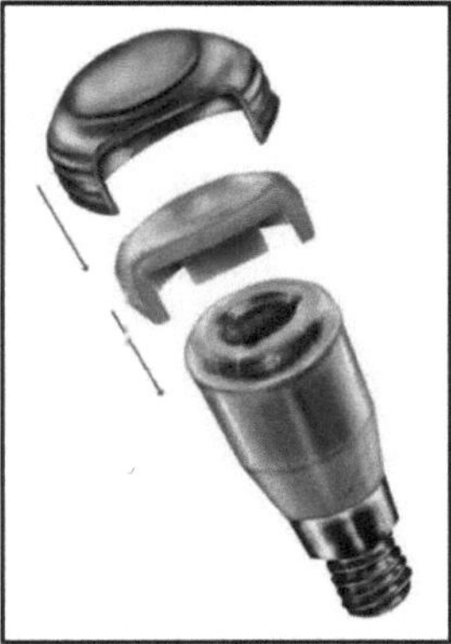

Figure 2: The different components of the Locator attachment(23)

The advantages of the LOCATOR attachment :

This system makes it possible to :

■Choose a retention adapted to the clinical situation thanks to the different retention inserts.

■Greater retention surface area than other systems thanks to double retention: internal and external.

■Reduce the risk of wear, as self-alignment will prevent incorrect insertion by the patient.

■Reduce the risk of retention loss thanks to nylon-titanium friction:

The nylon insert is in static contact with the abutment, while the metal capsule surrounding it can perform a stress-absorbing rotational movement.

■Guarantee a small footprint in clinical situations where space is at a premium.

available is reduced.

■Support divergences of up to 40° between two implants.

Finally, this attachment is compatible with several implant systems, with a relatively simple installation protocol for the practitioner or prosthetist and easy maintenance for the patient. (1)

Comparison between the LOCATOR attachment and the ball attachment:
Despite the historical success of the ball attachment for decades, the arrival of LOCATOR attachments on the dental implant market has transformed the ball attachment into an older retention complement.(23) (66)

Based on the results of a systematic review carried out in 2023 comparing LOCATOR attachment to axial ball attachment, the following conclusions were reached:

■LOCATOR attachment presents fewer complications

biomechanical: it can be used with a reduced inter-occlusal space, with a low risk of fracture. Less loss of retention has been observed.

■LOCATOR attachment presents fewer complications

and periodontium and less marginal bone loss.

■There was no significant difference between these two systems. in terms of the patient's overall satisfaction with the treatment.

❖Conjunction bars

Conjunction bars are used to secure the abutments and reduce the stress on them during prosthetic movements. The size and shape of the bars are dictated by the space available, the shape of the crest and the type of prosthesis.(23) Retention is by means of riders (short or long, made of metal or plastic) which are clipped onto the bar profile or by snap fasteners. (1)

There are different models of bars:

■The Acker Mann bar (spherical).
■The Dolder bar (ovoid or U-shaped) (fig.3)
■Hader bar (keyhole).

■The milled bar produced by casting, electroerosion or CAD/CAM. (fig.4).(36)

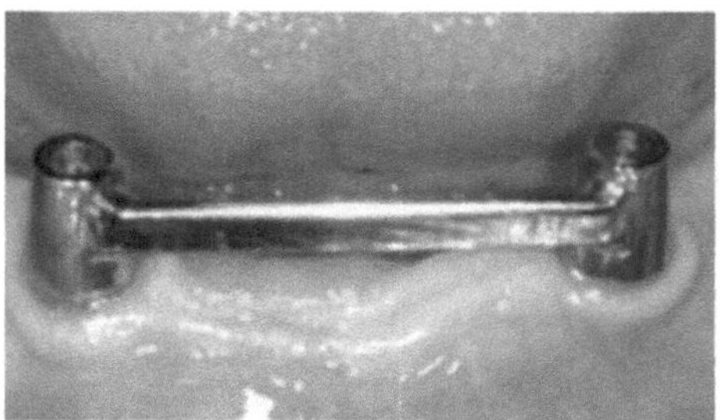

Figure 3: Bar connecting two implants(37).

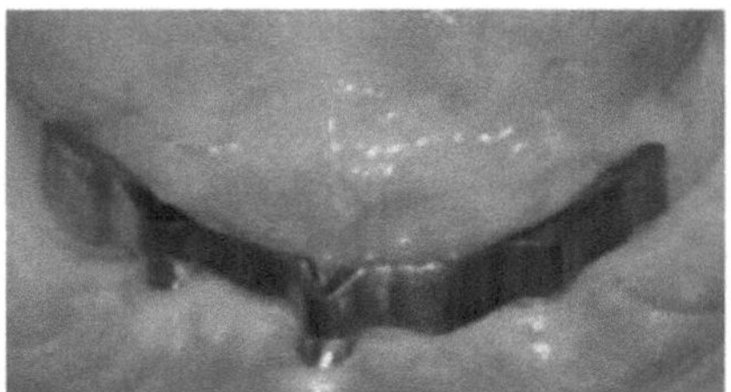

Figure 4: Milled bar machined using CAD/CAM

❖**Criteria for choosing an attachment system (61) (23) (1) (36) (15)**

•**Arcade concerned:** The survival rates for maxillary PACSI are lower than those for mandibular PACSI. Maxillary bone is spongy with a thin cortical layer, which influences osseointegration. In order to avoid failure, it is recommended that 4 to 6 implants be attached to the maxilla using a connector bar. In the mandible, the number of implants is 2 to 4, allowing the support of axial attachments or conjunction bars.

•**Shape of the ridge:** The choice of a connecting bar between two implants is indicated if the ridge is rectilinear. If the ridge is curvilinear, the prosthesis will protrude into the lingual region, causing significant functional discomfort, which is why axial attachments or segmented connector bars are preferred. The same applies to rounded or ogival ridges.

•**Available prosthetic space:** Conjunction bars require a large inter-head space (10mm), unlike axial attachments (6 to 8mm). The Locator system is one of the smallest retention systems available.

•**Implant parallelism:** Lack of implant parallelism can be compensated for by a conjunction bar or angulation-adjusting axial attachments. The parasitic forces resulting from this lack of parallelism cause wear to the attachment systems and even a loss of osseointegration.

•**Bone resorption and quality:** We recommend increasing the number of implants and securing them with a connecting bar in cases of unfavourable bone support.

•**Inter-implant distance:** For the design of a conjunction bar, the maximum distance between two implants is 15 mm to avoid deformation of the bar. Axial attachments are preferred to cantilever bars, which are contraindicated.

•**Processing cost :** The cost of axial attachments is relatively lower than that of the components required to produce a joint bar.

•**Implant loading :** If implants are to be loaded immediately to ensure primary stability, a splint is required.

1-1-2- Complete removable supra-implant prosthesis with telescopic crowns

The prosthesis is retained by friction. The telescopic system

is made up of secondary crowns attached to the prosthetic intrados (fig.5), which are fitted onto primary crowns (implant abutments) (fig.6). Primary crowns are classified according to their shapeand the orientation of their walls: a distinction is made between resilient, cylindrical or conical crowns (24) The results of a 10-year clinical and radiological follow-up study show that resilient telescopic crowns with two symphyseal implants appear to be an effective long-term treatment modality for edentulous and severely resorbed mandibles (26).

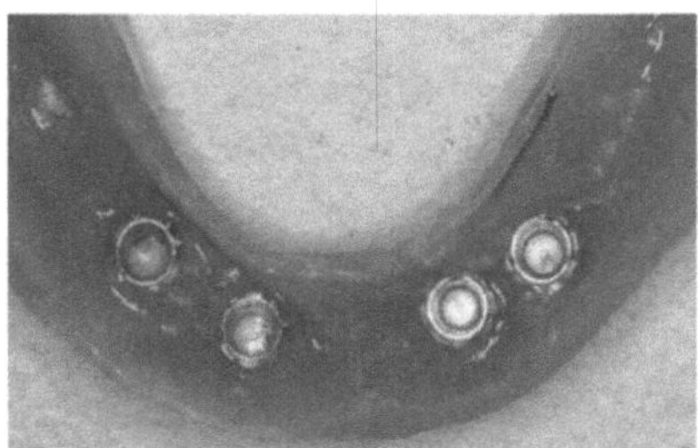

Figure 5: Prosthetic intrados with secondary crowns (29)

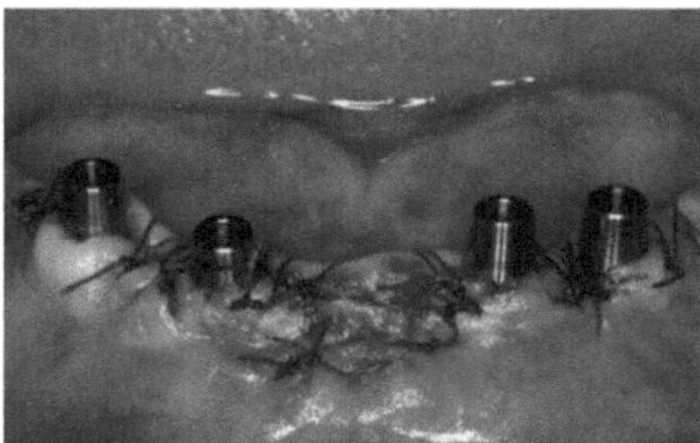

Figure 6: Primary crowns (implant abutments)(29)

1-2- Removable and non-removable solution

Complete removable supra-implant prosthesis with bar/counter-bar or non-removable screw-retained prosthesis or "removable bridge" It consists of a milled bar screwed onto implants and a counter-bar forming part of the prosthetic intrados. The removable part is held in place by friction: the prosthesis is fitted onto the bar using "snaps" to ensure retention. Cleats are found on the prosthetic extrados for fixation. (fig.7) The prosthesis is removable but the system has a certain rigidity which makes it similar to a fixed prosthesis. (6) Despite a high failure rate, if a removable supra-implant prosthesis is chosen for the maxilla, the use of a rigid bar (bar/counter-bar type) on a minimum of four non-aligned implants is recommended. This design minimises unfavourable biomechanical constraints. (39)

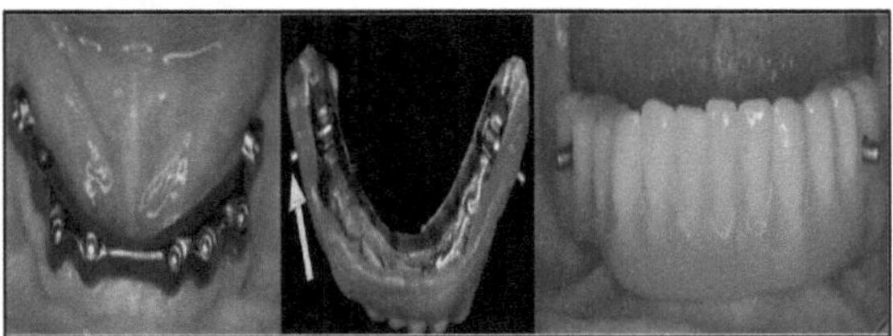

Figure 7: Non-removable mandibular screw-retained prosthesis supported by 6 implants: from left to right: bar tried in the mouth, prosthetic intrados showing the counter-bar and fixing lugs (yellow arrow) prosthesis in the mouth (36).

1-3- Fixed solution

1-3-1- The complete implant-supported bridge

The implant-supported full bridge is the solution that m o s t closely resembles natural anatomy. The height of the prosthetic teeth alone ensures that function and aesthetics are restored without the need for false gingiva. The prosthetic structure can be cemented or screw-retained onto implant abutments. (Fig.8) This type of prosthesis is chosen in cases where the available prosthetic space has been reduced and to meet the patient's requirements for a fixed solution.

Ideally, in the maxilla, the prosthesis is sectioned into four 3-unit bridges with a supporting implant at each end of the bridge. This method requires 8 implants and can support 12 prosthetic teeth. In the mandible, it is generally considered that 4 to 6 implants are sufficient for this form of reconstruction, the difference in the number of implants being due to the distribution of the implants and bone density (51).

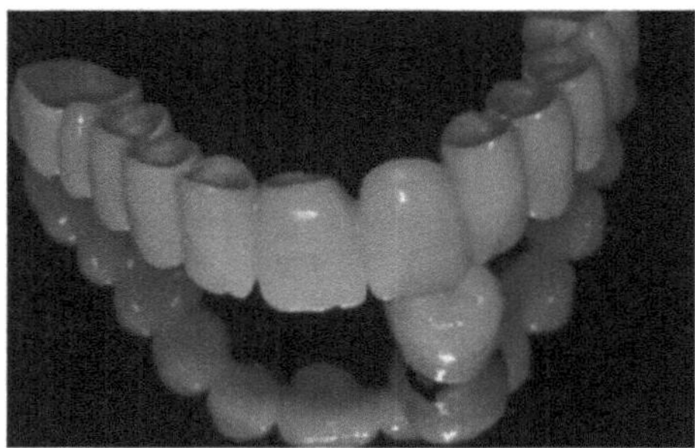

Figure 8: Implant-supported full bridge(69)

1-3-2- Brånemark bridge or bridge "on stilts" The name "on stilts" comes from the fact that the prosthesis does not touch the edentulous ridge. ridge. It is a prosthesis screw-retained on 4 or 6 implants. (fig.9)The BRÂNEMARK type has the longest clinical follow-up (30 years) (67) (44).

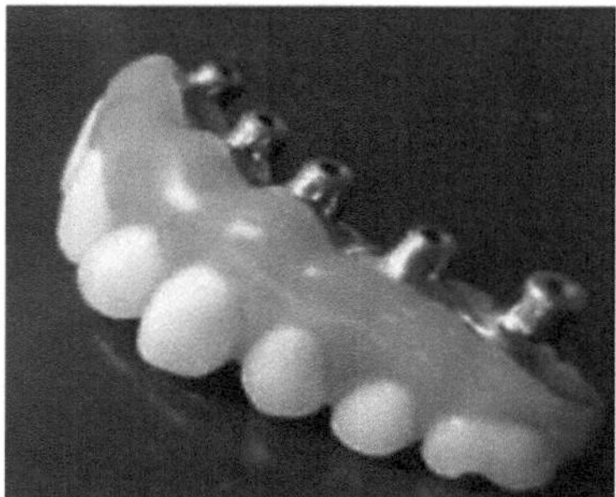

Figure 9: Bridge on piles (67)

1-3-3- Hybrid prosthesis screwed onto implants

The hybrid prosthesis lies between the implant-supported full bridge and the bridge on posts. It features an intermediate structure to compensate for the mismatch between the emergences of the implant abutments and the prosthetic teeth. It comprises a framework screwed onto the implant abutments, onto which a counter-frame is cemented.The counter framework can be divided into several elements (fig.10) in order to meet aesthetic and biomechanical requirements. It consists of teeth and false gingiva (37) (25) (66) (48) A metal framework can also be designed on which prosthetic teeth can be mounted (fig.11).

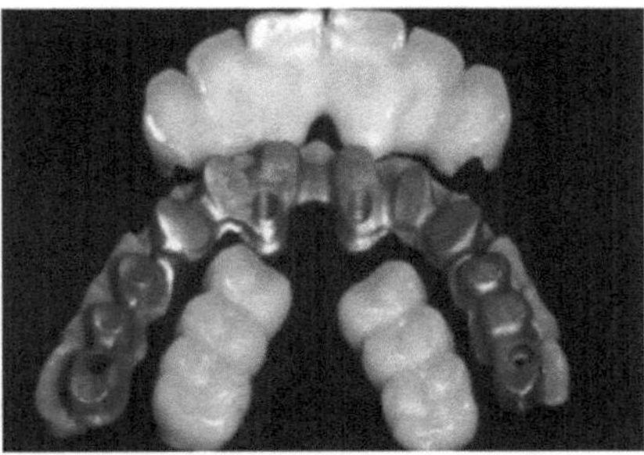

Figure 10: Hybrid prosthesis with a counterpart divided into 3 counterframes(32)

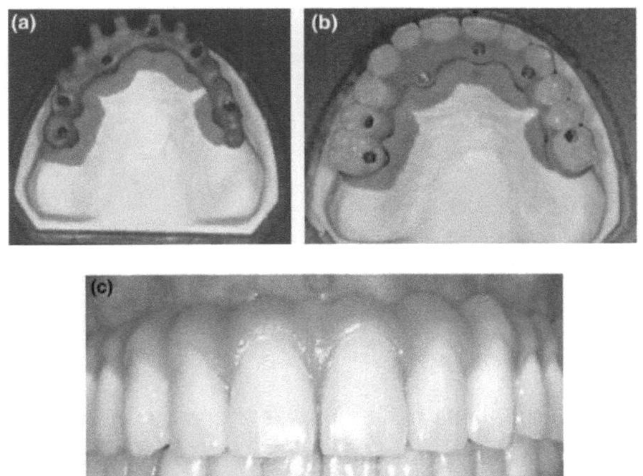

Figure 11: Maxillary screw-retained hybrid prosthesis assembled on 6 implants: (a) titanium framework machined using CAD/CAM. (b) fitting of prosthetic teeth (c) final aesthetic result (37)

1-4- Number and distribution of implants according to the type of supra-implant restoration in the edentulous patient

1-4-1- For a removable restoration

❖ Maxillary

The results of a retrospective study in 2009 support the concept of PACSI treatment in the maxilla, provided that a minimum of 4 non-aligned implants are placed and secured with a bar (52). (Fig 12-13) Data on minimal designs with fewer than 4 implants in the maxilla are rare and have shown significantly poorer results(28).

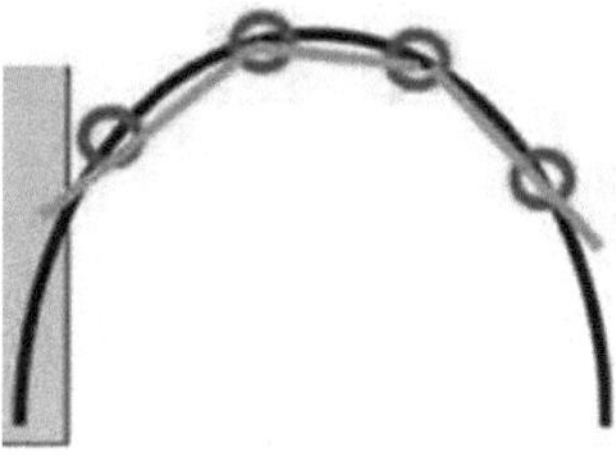

Figure 12: Maxillary screw-retained hybrid prosthesis assembled on 6 implants: (a) titanium framework machined using CAD/CAM. (b) fitting of prosthetic teeth.(c) final aesthetic result.(37)

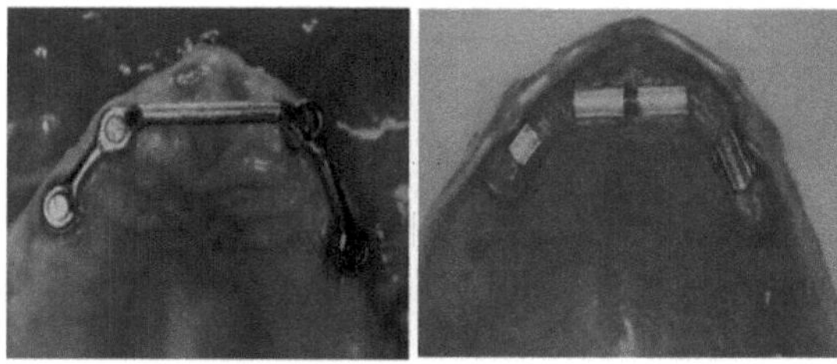

Figure 13: Maxillary PACSI with 4 non-aligned implants secured by a bar: A: bar tried in the mouth. B: prosthetic intrados with riders (32)

❖ **At the mandible**

The placement of two implants for a removable prosthesis in the mandible gave favourable results. However, it should be noted that four implants have shown slightly better results. The number of implants depends on the shape of the arch (fig 14) (28).

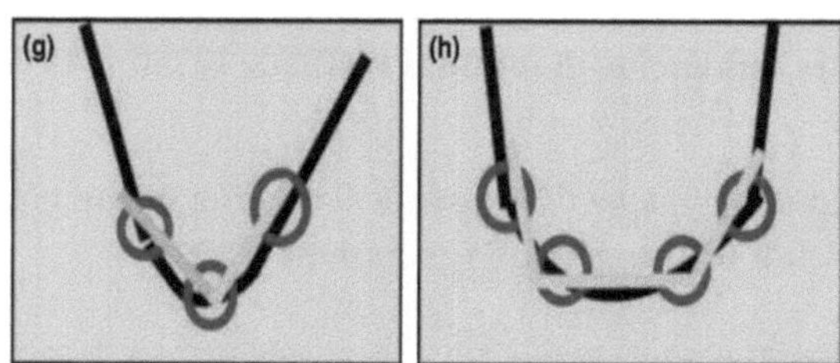

Figure 14: Graphic illustrations: depending on the shape of the mandibular arch (V-shaped or rectangular), a number of 3 or 4 implants is suggested. The bar segments should be 15 mm long(37).

1-4-2- For fixed reconstruction

❖ Maxillary

The placement of six or more implants in the maxilla gives favourable results (fig.15). If we consider the "all-on-4" concept for the maxilla, the study by Crespi et al. in 2012 reveals satisfactory results with acceptable evidence. (28)

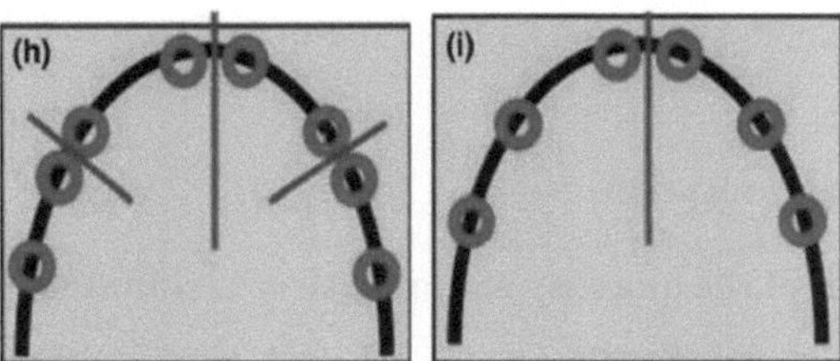

Figure 15: Graphic illustrations: Distribution of 6-8 implants and segmentation possibilities for the metal frame(37)

❖ At the mandible

The use of 4 to 6 implants is a well-documented treatment option giving satisfactory results. (55,27). In addition, four implants with a removable prosthesis had a better result than four implants with a fixed prosthesis in the mandible(28).

CHAPTER 2

**DECISION-MAKING CRITERIA FOR SUPRA-IMPLANT
RESTORATIONS IN THE FULLY EDENTULOUS PATIENT**

The success of supra-implant prosthetic treatment depends on reasoned and comprehensive planning based on a set of criteria.

2-1- The degree of resorption

2-1-1- Assessment of the quantity and quality of residual bone

Favourable bone support ensures the success of implant treatment, but the practitioner is often faced with clinical situations where bone quality and quantity are affected. (fig.16) In the completely edentulous patient, resorption occurs following tooth loss.

This post-extraction resorption can reach 50% of the total bone volume after one year. Resorption is centripetal in the maxilla and centrifugal in the mandible (with the exception of the anterior incisor region)(56).

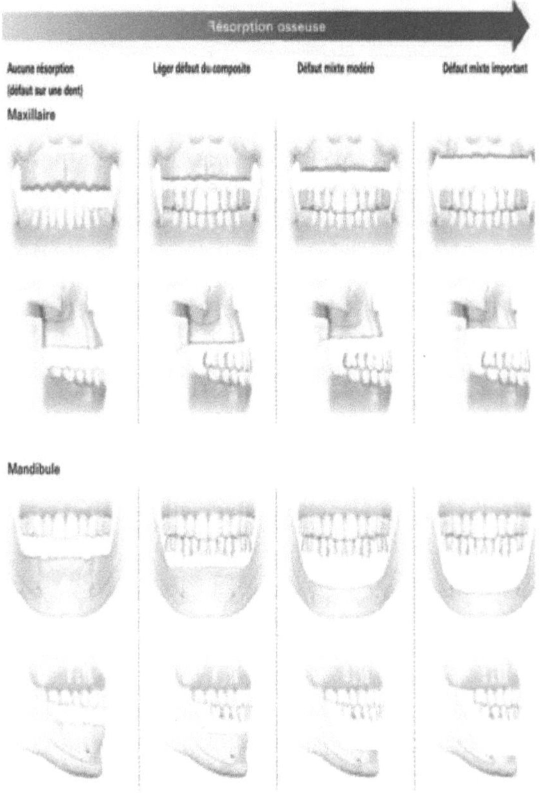

Figure 16: Volume of hard and soft tissue loss following complete edentulism of the arches. (68)

Several classifications have been proposed to assess the condition of edentulous ridges receiving future implant sites and supra-implant prostheses. Based on the volume of bone available, Cawood and Howell proposed a pathophysiological classification consisting of six stages describing the alveolar resorption of edentulous ridges:

■Class I: toothed.

■Class II: post-extraction.

■Class III: rounded crest: sufficient height and width.

■Class IV: knife-edge ridge: sufficient height, insufficient width.

■Class V: flat crest: insufficient height and width.

■Class VI: concave crest (with loss of basal bone)(56) (fig.17)

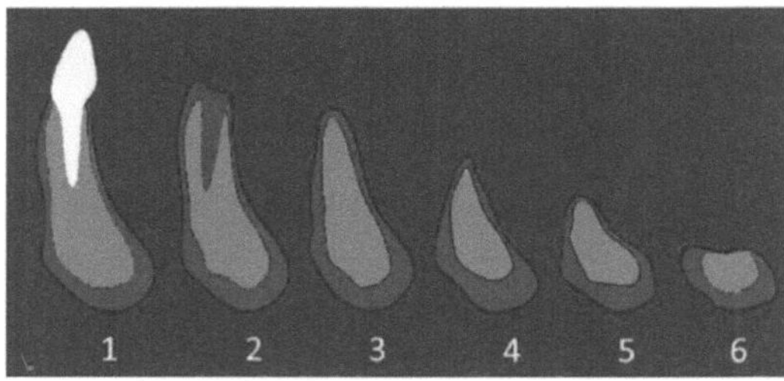

Figure 17: Stages of bone resorption according to Cawood and Howell(56)

The Lekholm and Zarb classification, which dates back to 1985, is based on bone density and the distribution between cortical and cancellous bone tissue to differentiate the bone quality of the sites to be implanted. This classification guides the choice of the type of implants used as well as the implant site preparation protocol (drilling) in order to obtain sufficient primary stability, which is essential for the long-term success of the implant treatment (59).

A distinction is made between :

▪ Type I bone: dense bone composed entirely of compact bone.
▪ Type II bone: a thick layer of compact bone surrounding a core o f   cancellous bone.
▪ Type III bone: a thin layer of compact bone which surrounds a core of cancellous bone: the cancellous part is densely trabeculated, giving it a

good resistance.

▪ Type IV bone: a thin layer of compact bone surrounding a core of bone

spongy: the predominant spongy part is of low density causing low resistance. (Fig.18) (56)

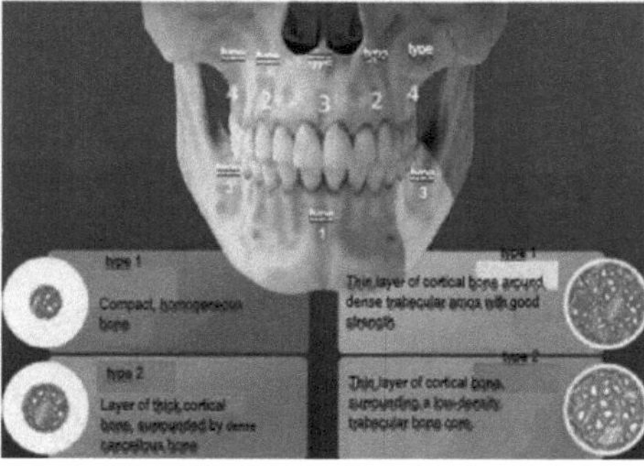

Figure 18: Distribution of different bone types in the maxilla and mandible (70)

These authors also described 5 stages of resorption based on bone volume:

■Class A: most of the alveolar crest is present " bone without resorption".

■Class B: moderate resorption of the alveolar ridge.

■Class C: significant resorption of the alveolar ridge.

■Class D: onset of basal bone resorption.

■Class E: extreme resorption of basal bone (fig.19)

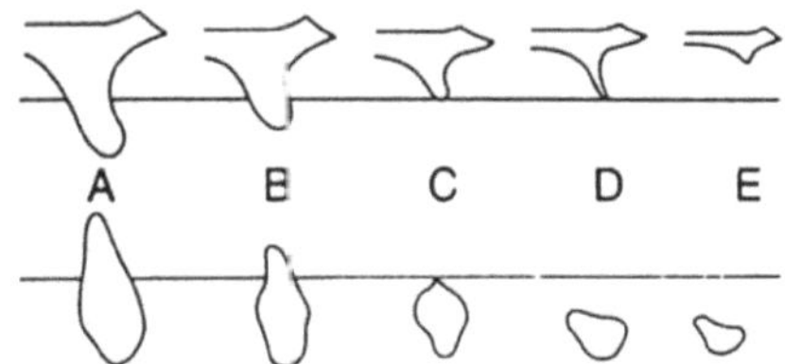

Figure 19: Classification of bone resorption according to Zarb and Lekholm (19)

If major bone surgery is refused, it is essential to optimise the use of residual bone volumes in order to guarantee the success of implant treatment without grafting in the totally edentulous patient(43).The more advanced the resorption of completely edentulous ridges, the more rational it would be to opt for prosthetic restorations that make preferential use of the premaxilla and mandibular symphysis. It is the amount of bone available in these areas that guides the choice of the type of implants used, their positions and the surgical technique adopted, as well as the implant restoration indicated.

2-1-2- Evaluation of the available prosthetic space (EPD)

The patient may present with different types of atrophy. Quantifying the degree of tissue loss is a key point, as resorption may occur vertically, horizontally, or both, which is difficult to recognise. EPD assessment is used to quantify the degree of vertical resorption. The available restorative space is measured from the implant neck to the incisal edge in the anterior region and to the occlusal plane in the posterior region, and it is this space that will determine the choice of prosthesis(62). The authors have classified this space into 4 categories (44): (fig.20)

■D1: minimal (10-12 mm).

■D2: moderate (12-15 mm).

■D3: moderate (15-18 mm).

∎D4: excessive (>18mm).

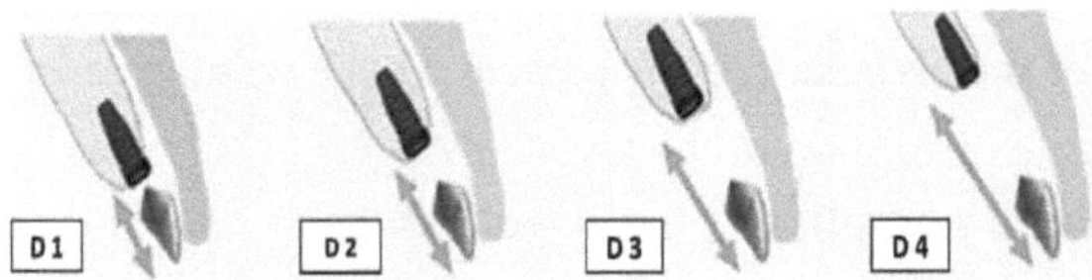

Figure 20: Space available between the implant neck and the incisal edge or occlusal plane of the future prosthetic teeth (62)

The choice of type of prosthesis and final restorative material depends on the space available. (Table 1) (62)If the space available is relatively limited, a full implant-supported bridge is the most appropriate treatment. However, if the space between the ridge and the opposite arch is increased, the prosthesis must replace the soft tissues as well as the teeth, hence the use of a false gum.(30) Similarly, the technical success of prosthetic materials depends on certain minimum space requirements that must be met. If prosthetic materials are used in thinner sections, there will be more failures related to fracture of the prosthesis. (62)

Table 1: Prosthetic alternatives according to available prosthetic space. (62)

Distance inter-crête (Plateforme de l'implant /crête jusqu'à la dentition opposée)	Type des prothèses
1 10-12mm	**Solution fixe** Bridge complet implanto-porté (céramo-métallique /céramo-céramique : zircone monolithique ou zircone stratifiée) **Solution amovible** contre-indiquée
2 12-15mm	**Solution fixe** Bridge complet implanto-porté (céramo-métallique / céramo-céramique zircone monolithique ou zircone stratifiée) Avec une fausse gencive **Solution amovible** PACSI avec attachements de type LOCATOR ou des couronnes télescopiques Les barres sont contre indiquées.
3 15-18 mm	**Solution fixe** armature métallique et montage des dents en résine acrylique armature bio-HPP (Biocompatible High Performance Polymer) et montage des dents en résine composite Armature fraisée et vissée sur laquelle sont scellés des couronnes ou des bridges de petite étendue **Solution amovible** PACSI avec des attachements Locator ou boule ou couronnes télescopiques ou barre fraisée à profil bas
4 >18 mm	**Solution fixe** Contre-indiquée **Solution amovible** PACSI avec une barre fraisée ou coulée ou couronnes télescopiques

The notion of available prosthetic space also applies to the choice of retention complement for PACSI: the use of a conjunction bar requires more prosthetic space than for axial attachments. (Table 2) (60)

Table 2: Recommended space for different types of attachment systems. (47)

Recommended space	Conventional prosthesis	Locator	Ball	Milled bar	Clip-on bar and jumpers
Acrylic resin	>2-3mm	>3mm	>3mm	>3mm	>3mm
The Implant Abutment	-	1.5 mm	>3.7 mm	>5mm +2mm Of gingival clearance	Dolder :>3-5mm+ >2mm of gingival clearance Hader : >4.5mm+2mm of gingival clearance
The retentive retentive element (sub-prosthetic)	-	3.2 mm	>2.4 mm	-	Dolder: >3-4 mm Hader: >2.5 mm
Occlusal space required	>3mm	>8-9 mm + 1mm In case bruxism	>9 mm + 1 mm in case of bruxism	>10mm +1mm for bruxism	>12mm + 1mm in case of bruxism
Vestibulo-lingual width required	>3mm	10 mm	10 mm	-	11mm
Vestibular and lingual width required from the centre of the implant screw	-	3mm	4 mm	-	4mm

2-2-Aesthetic requirements

Treatment of the edentulous jaw poses a number of problems, complicated by the fact that the loss of teeth and bone affects the harmony of the face. Expectations regarding the aesthetics of the final prosthesis can be high. (5) Edentulous patients may have virtually intact alveolar bone volume and only missing clinical crowns, or they may have alveolar bone resorption and soft tissue loss requiring the use of a false gingiva to compensate for this defect(5).

▶ **Bone support defects in the maxilla and repercussions on aesthetics :**

In the maxilla, in cases of Zarb and Lekholm stages A or B bone resorption **(fig.19),** the existing bone volume does not compromise the final aesthetic result. However, from stage C onwards, a choice must be made between longer teeth or the use of prosthetic false gingiva or bone grafts to meet the aesthetic imperative. (49) Depending on the degree of bone resorption, a type of prosthetic rehabilitation will be suggested:

■Low bone resorption: fixed prosthesis that does not contain a false tooth gingiva (screwed or cemented).

■Medium resorption : Fixed prosthesis with false gum (screwed or cemented)

■Significant bone loss: a removable prosthesis (overdenture) on a bar(31) **(fig.21)**

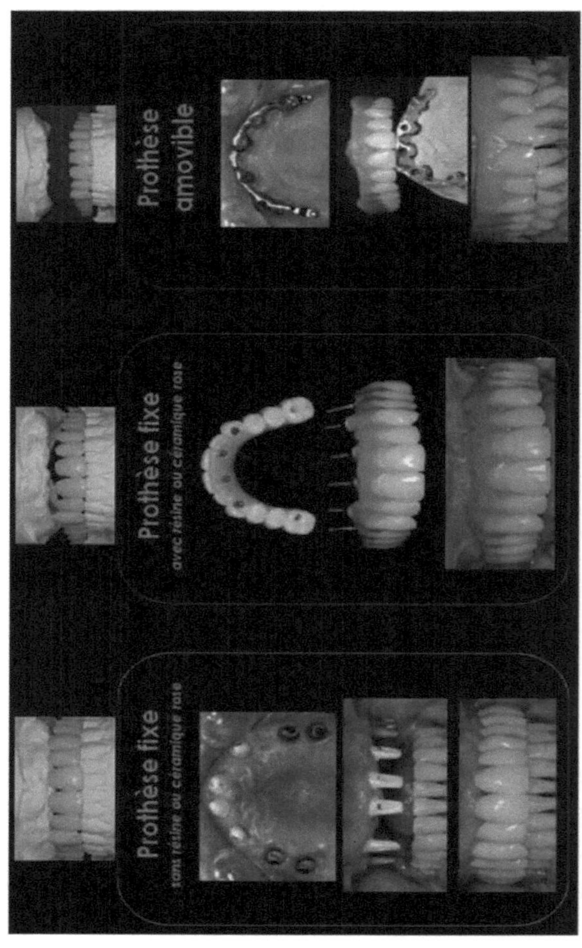

Figure 21: Prosthetic rehabilitation proposals according to the bone support defect to restore aesthetics (31)

Aesthetic parameters influencing the choice of supra-implant prosthesis :

• Smile line :

It corresponds to the position of the edge of the vermilion of the upper lip in relation to the visible part of the teeth and gums. The degree of visibility of the residual ridge is assessed at the moment of maximum smile without any retractor. (5)

Tjan et al. have established a classification of the smile according to the degree of visibility of the teeth and gum tissue:

■ The low smile line: exposure of less than 75% of the teeth before.

■ The average smile line: movements of the lips uncover between 75 and 100% of the front teeth and the gum line.interproximal.

■ The high smile line: the smile fully exposes the front teeth and a strip of gum (62).

Recent studies have distinguished a fourth type of smile: the "gingival smile", defined as total exposure of the anterior teeth and exposure of more than 3 to 4 mm of gingival tissue. (fig.22)(8)

The relationship between the smile line and the appearance of the prosthesis must be taken into consideration in any complete maxillary rehabilitation.

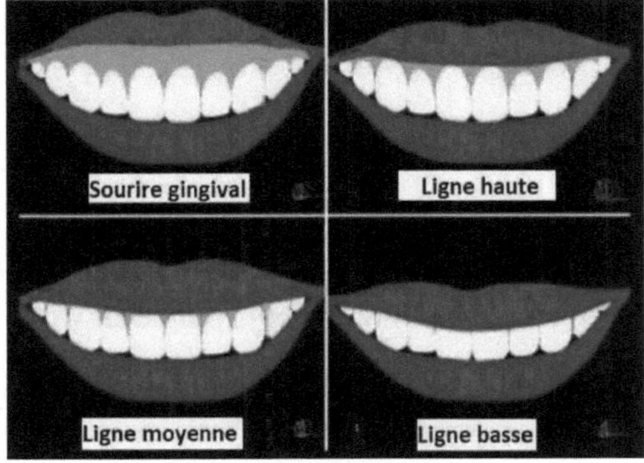

Figure 22: Different types of smile line (18)

• Transition line :

This is an imaginary line that marks the boundary between the residual crest and the most apical part of the future prosthesis. (40) The final aesthetic result depends on the position of the transition line in relation to the smile line.

If the patient has a low smile line that does not allow the ridge to be seen, the transition between the prosthesis and the residual soft tissue does not involve any aesthetic risk. An implant-supported full bridge is then of interest. (**fig 23 and 25**) . On the other hand, if the smile line is high and the residual ridge is visible, the aesthetic compromise will be high, and the lost tissue will have to be replaced in addition to the teeth. There is a choice between a fixed implant-supported prosthesis with false gingiva or a removable supra-implant prosthesis (**fig.24 and 26**). The replacement of lost dento-osseous elements is carried out using a prosthetic false gum which will guarantee alignment of collars, aesthetic interdental papillae and appropriate dental proportions. (30) (40)

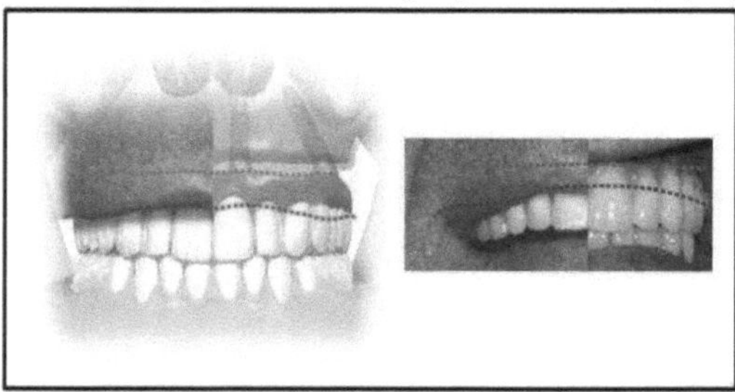

Figure 23: Apical transition line (green) compared with the smile line (red): aesthetic result (68).

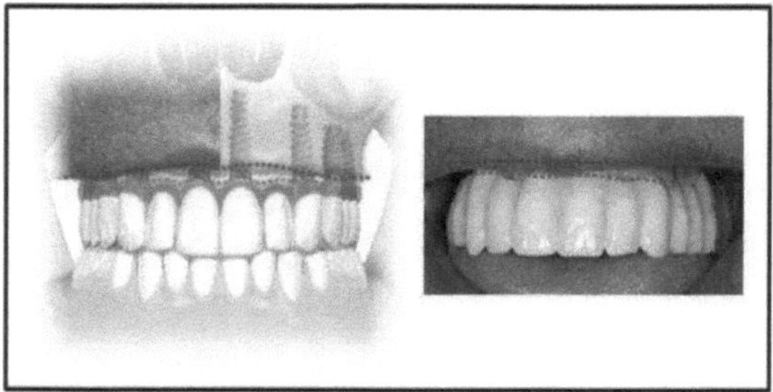

Figure 24: Coronal transition line (green) compared with the smile line (red): unsightly result(68).

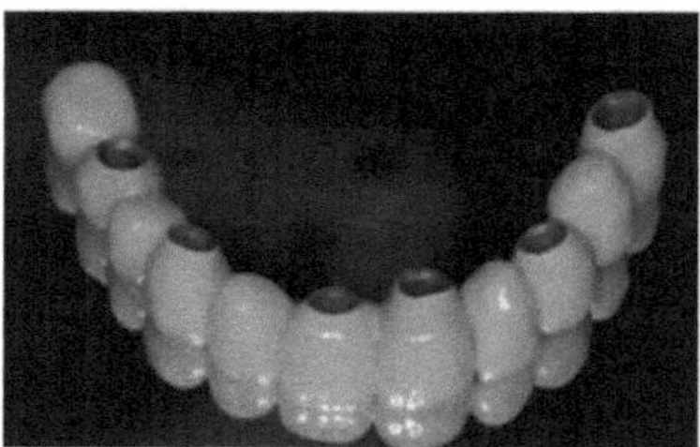

Figure 25: Implant-supported bridge without false gingiva(4)

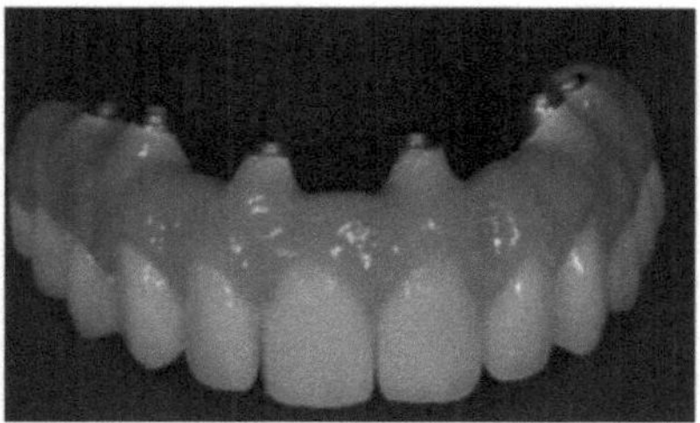

Figure 26: Bridge on posts with false gingiva(4).

• The position of the incisal edge :

It is essential to determine the ideal position of this margin on the face, as it helps to determine aesthetics, the occlusal plane and the vertical occlusal dimension. Its ideal position is determined by aesthetics and phonetics. It is conventionally established that the occlusal plane for the completely edentulous patient, parallel to the bi-pupillary plane at the anterior level, lies 2mm below the lower edge of the upper lip (40).

• Position of the cervical margin and position of the incisors in relation to the ridge :

Once the position of the maxillary incisal edge has been determined, the length of the incisors can be established using standard dental proportions, the patient's anterior dental casts or aesthetically acceptable photographs (40) (9). The height and width of the prosthetic teeth should be based on aesthetic dental proportions and not on the location of the patient's anterior residual ridge. If there is additional space between the aesthetically determined neck of the prosthetic teeth and the ridge, it should be filled with an aesthetic prosthetic material that simulates the gingival tissues. The false gum(40) (9)

• Lip support :

The static and dynamic positions of the upper lip and its tone are determining factors when deciding on the type of prosthesis and the resulting aesthetics. The dentition and bone volume of the premaxilla provide support for the upper lip (15). (fig.27) But the perception of lip support depends on a number of variables: the amount of resorption of the alveolar bone, the thickness of the lips, which varies according to age, sex and race, the length of the nose, the morphology of the cartilaginous part of the lower nose, the nasal septum, the anterior nasal spine, the tip of the nose, the nasolabial angle, the projection of the chin and facial hair (the moustache and beard in men)(8).

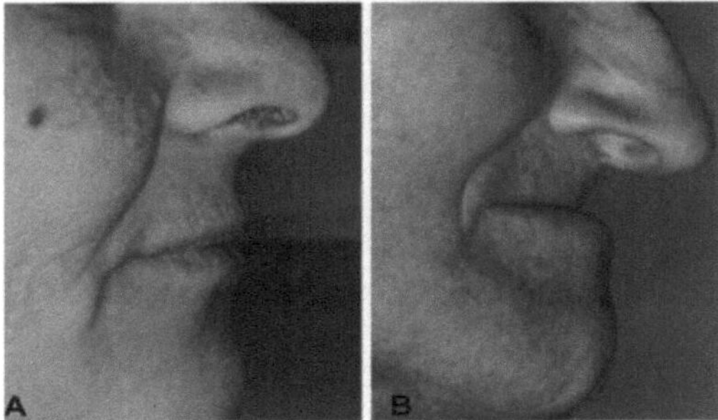

Figure 27: Restoration of lip support (A) / loss of lip support (30)

If the patient does not require labial support, a fixed prosthesis is indicated; however, if labial support is required, a removable prosthesis is preferred(30). Patient approval of labial support is crucial at the diagnostic stage as patients with severe resorption who are dissatisfied with their appearance may reconsider the option of an implant-supported removable prosthesis as the thickness of the anterior labial margin may better meet their aesthetic needs. (Fig 28) (8)

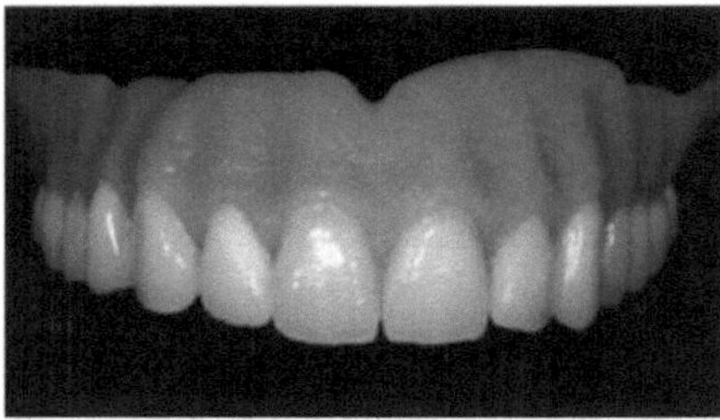

Figure 28:Removable supra-implant total prosthesis with an extended anterior labial margin to support the lip (4)

However, if the patient is going to benefit from a fixed implant-supported restoration in the edentulous maxilla, a series of elements need to be analysed (the smile line, the transition line between the residual ridge and the prosthesis, the labial support, the position of the incisal edges and the necks of the teeth, the proportions of the prosthetic teeth) in order to meet the aesthetic requirements of the future prosthesis. A study carried out in 2010 by Bidra et al. reported that patients were classified into 4 groups in order to identify the need or otherwise for a false gum and labial support: One of the major differences between the classes is the prosthetic space available, which decreases progressively from class I to class IV. The Class IV patient is distinguished by being the only one to present a high smile line or a "gingival" smile, exposing a large part of the residual ridge. (9)Table 3 and the diagram (fig 29) explain in detail the conclusions reached.

Table 3: Diagnosis of the elements involved in the classification of Bidra et al.(9)

Patient classification	Loss of tissue	Position of the anterior teeth in relation to the anterosuperior ridge	Position of the smile line in relation to the denture-junction residual peak	Need for false gums
I	Severe to moderate	Lower and front	Incisal	The false gingiva ensures labial support and correct proportions of the teeth
II	Moderate	Lower	Insicale	The false gum ensures correct proportions of teeth only
II	Minimal or absent	On the ridge directly	Insicale	Not recommended
IV	There is an excess of fabrics	Surgical intervention required	Apical	Dependson the new class after intervention

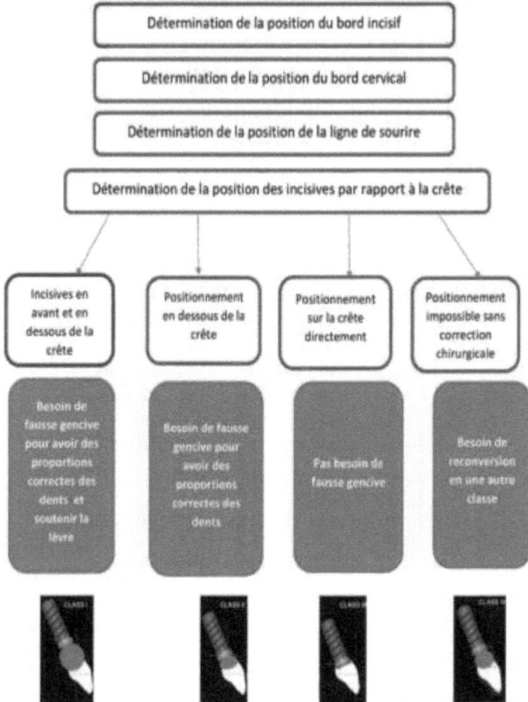

Figure 29: Aesthetic classification of edentulous patients for rehabilitation with a fixed maxillary prosthesis. (8) (9)

2-3- Inter-peak ratio

Based on the principle that the forces exerted by an implant should be oriented as far as possible along its axis, it seems essential to determine the skeletal class (fig.30), especially when there is resorption. which determines the three-dimensional placement of implants over the entire arch (49).

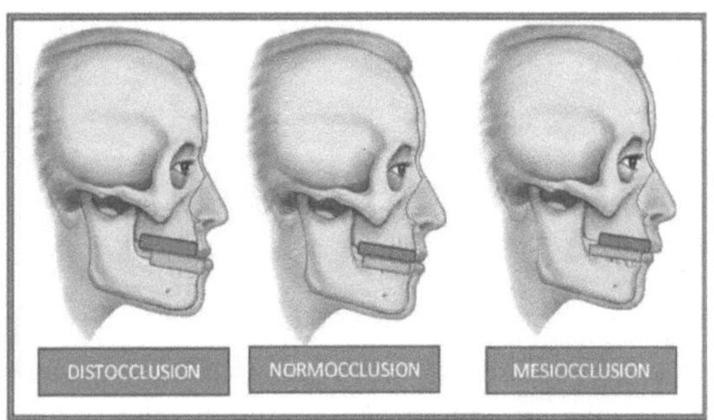

Figure 30: Different inter-ridge ratios in the fully edentulous patient. (41)

■If a "NORMOCCLUSION" class is present, the treatment option is determined according to the residual bone volume (49).

■The "MESIOCCLUSION" class corresponds to the very anterior position of the maxilla in relation to the mandible.

It is extremely complex to achieve palatal angulation of maxillary anterior implants and vestibular angulation of mandibular implants. It can lead to a reduction in lip stability and/or a significant change in facial appearance, which may be difficult for the patient to tolerate. It is necessary to consider prosthetic compensation for the offset of the bases.In the maxilla, a significant difference between the bone bases is a major contraindication to the use of a supra-implant fixed prosthesis. In these unfavourable conditions, a fixed implant-prosthetic rehabilitation will result in a horizontal overhang, an ineffective anterior guide, disturbed phonation and overcontouring of the dental morphology in order to guarantee minimal aesthetics(16). In the mandible, where there is a significant offset, a full implant-supported bridge will result in an anterior gap. The presence of a moderate offset can be compensated for by a more anterior angulation of the symphyseal implants(49).

■The "DISTOCCLUSION" class: refers to the posterior position of the maxilla in relation to the mandible.

In the maxilla, where bone volume is favourable, a more vestibular angulation of the implants and an appropriate prosthetic design can reduce or even rectify the skeletal offset. In the mandible, where there is a large volume of bone, lingual angulation of the implants and an appropriate prosthetic design can reduce or even rectify the skeletal misalignment. When bone volume is reduced, it is not recommended to use a fixed implant prosthesis in the maxilla or mandible (49). For example, PACSI can be useful for patients with excessively misaligned mesial or distal bone base ratios. Whereas bridge

The "on stilts" or fixed implant-supported prosthesis is only recommended for NORMO or MESIOCLUSION class cases. The full implant-supported bridge is only recommended in cases where the inter-crestal ratio is favourable. (16)

2-4-Antagonist arcade

The natural dentition or the type of prosthesis present in the opposite arch will have an impact on the choice of supra-implant rehabilitation. Based on a certain hypothesis, when the antagonist arch is dentate or fitted with a fixed implant-supported prosthesis and there is a risk of para-functional activity (nocturnal bruxism), the use of a PACSI is recommended because it can be removed during the night (20). With this in mind, a systematic review of the literature carried out in 2010 to study the impact of remaining natural teeth in the antagonist arch on implant survival and the success of implant-supported removable treatments (ISRPs) in the maxilla and mandible concluded that the presence of teeth in the antagonist arch does not present any risk for the success of mandibular ISRPs, whereas if the ISRP is maxillary, the presence of opposing teeth may constitute a risk factor but is not certainly a contraindication(45). Carayon et al. have suggested that the maxillary supra-implant complete removable prosthesis may be indicated if the antagonist's arch comprises either natural teeth, or a denture-supported or implant-supported fixed prosthesis, or a supra-implant removable prosthesis. This treatment is contraindicated if the antagonist is a conventional removable prosthesis, as it would lead to accelerated bone resorption and prosthetic instability, sometimes with fractures(12).

2-5- Health situation

For elderly patients (aged 50 and over) who may lack dexterity and/or have limited vision, patients suffering from systemic diseases with manual and rheumatological repercussions, and patients with poor oral hygiene, removable supra-implant prostheses may be preferable because they can be removed and are therefore easier to clean. This ability to easily remove the prosthesis is also a more favourable option for people with acquired or congenital maxillofacial defects, as it can be easily removed by the attending physician (oncologist) during medical consultations or in the event of complications.(20)

2-6- Cost and financial resources

Access to dental care is mainly hampered by cost. Insurance schemes have a positive impact on patients' attitudes and motivation to seek dental care(33). Over a period of 15 years, Attard et al. carried out an economic study of fixed and removable prostheses. Their results showed that treatment costs were significantly higher for the fixed prosthesis group, even when long-term results were taken into account. As a general rule, more implants are required to support fixed prostheses than for maintain a prosthesis removable therefore fixed rehabilitation can be more expensive than a removable rehabilitation. (38,20).

2-7- Patient preferences

Patient preference plays a crucial role in planning supra-implant treatments. These preferences arise from subjective, socio-economic and cultural factors such as personal perceptions, past experiences, attitudes and beliefs about prosthetic treatment and, in some cases, may simply be a personal decision. It should be noted that patient preference can potentially be related to social and financial status (33).

2-8-Technical and clinical skills of dentists and dental laboratory technicians

From a clinical point of view, the overall rehabilitation of fixed prostheses is complexon several levels: the complexity of the production methods (recording of occlusal ratios, precision of the impression on numerous implant preparations and abutments) and to obtain lasting functional stability with a satisfactory aesthetic result for the patient(7).From a technical point of view, despite advances in foundry techniques, the conventional prosthetic chain is subject to an accumulation of inaccuracies due to the nature of the materials used and their handling: the risk of errors associated with coating, the risk of deformation of the metal element and the non-homogeneity of the metal. For fixed implant-supported (hybrid) prostheses, it is much easier to obtain and reproduce the passivity of the frameworks by CAD/CAM and guarantee the quality of the result than by traditional casting techniques. Machining is the reference technique, and the use of subtraction machining and computer modelling techniques ensures that the material undergoes no structural modification. Implant suprastructures are also manufactured using CAD/CAM with the most precise prosthetic parts. But the use of CAD/CAM techniques requires the skills of prosthetists and practitioners, as well as dental laboratories and practices equipped with sophisticated digital equipment. (34)The clinical and technical production of implant-supported removable prostheses is therefore simpler than that of fixed implant-supported prostheses (20).

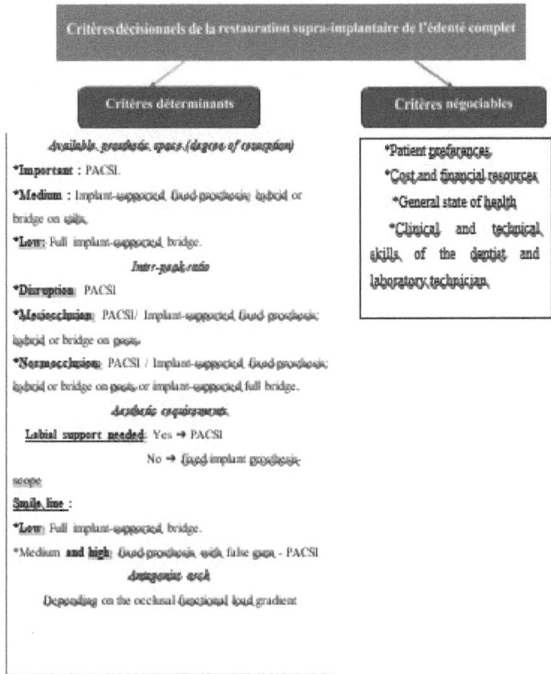

Figure 31: Decision-making criteria for the choice of prosthetic rehabilitation in the edentulous patient.

CHAPTER 3

PREOPERATIVE ASSESSMENT OF SUPRA-IMPLANT REHABILITATION IN THE EDENTULOUS PATIENT

The success of implant-supported prosthetic rehabilitation depends on a well-executed preoperative assessment that covers a number of elements, the most important of which are detailed below:

3-1- Photographs of the patient

Exo-buccal and endo-buccal photographs should be taken prior to treatment in order to record the patient's aesthetic characteristics and make comparisons during the different therapeutic phases(40).

3-2- Examination of the mouth opening and the temporomandibular joint (TMJ)

TMJ pathologies need to be diagnosed and the assessment of the the mouth opening is essential from the preoperative study phase, as the placement of implants in the posterior sectors requires a minimum mouth opening of 4 to 6 mm. This value may be higher if angled implants are used and guided or dynamic surgery is employed(40).

3-3- Articulator mounting

It is essential to record the occlusion during the study phase. The study models derived from the impressions, mounted on an articulator, enable analysis of the initial situation, the available prosthetic space, the inter-arch relationship and the occlusal parameters.

3-4-Evaluation of the available subprosthetic space

In the case of PACSI, the available prosthetic space must be evaluated by silicone keys to enable the various components of the axial attachments to be superimposed. (Fig. 32) The space will be different depending on the type of attachment planned, which is specific to each manufacturer. (47)

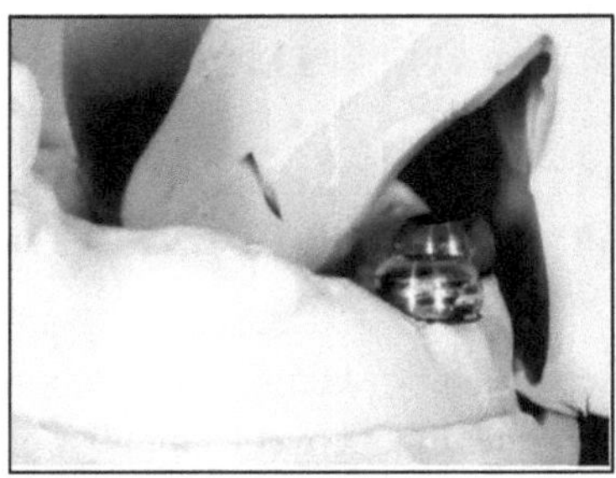

Figure 32: A sectioned silicone key used to measure the space around each Locator(47).

3-5- Assessment of aesthetic parameters

To analyse the aesthetic appearance of the prosthesis during the preoperative phase, a transparent resin duplicate of the prosthetic project **(fig.33)** can be made and tested in the mouth (42).

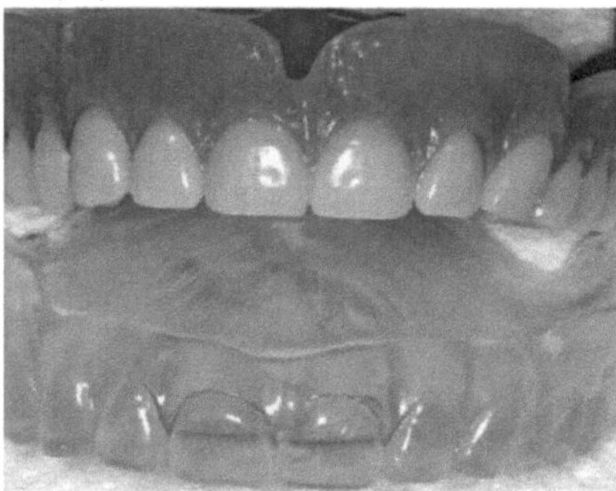

Figure 33: Duplicate prosthesis (40)

The papillae of the duplicate are marked in black before the duplicate is placed in the mouth to assess its aesthetic appearance (fig 34 and 35)(42).

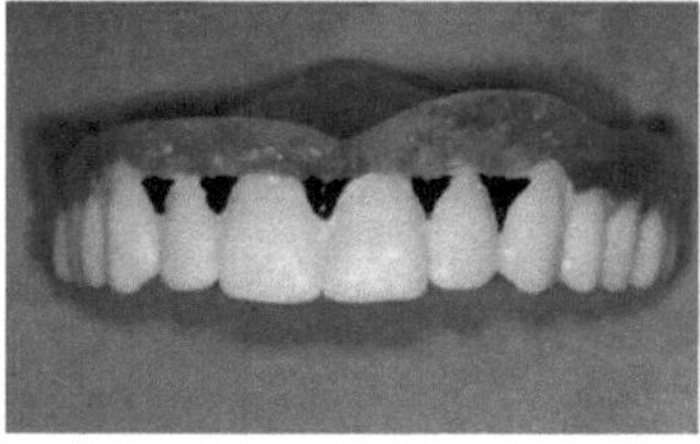

Figure 34: Papillae marked in black to assess the position of the smile line (42).

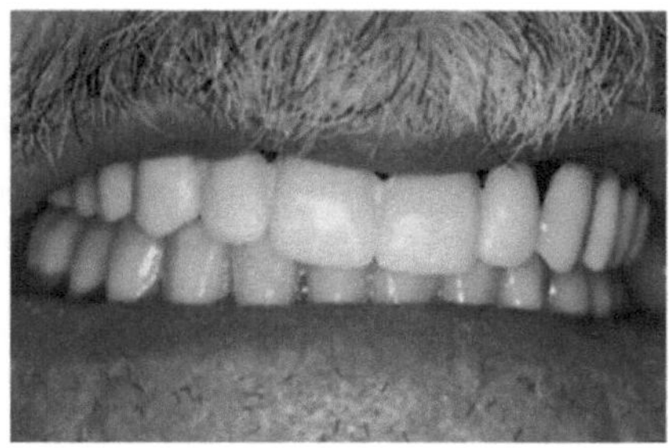

Figure 35: Frontal view with the duplicate in the mouth: the papillae are visible. (42).

The labial margin of the duplicate will be removed above the anterior teeth to determine the need for labial support without the benefit of this margin (fig. 36 and 37) (42).

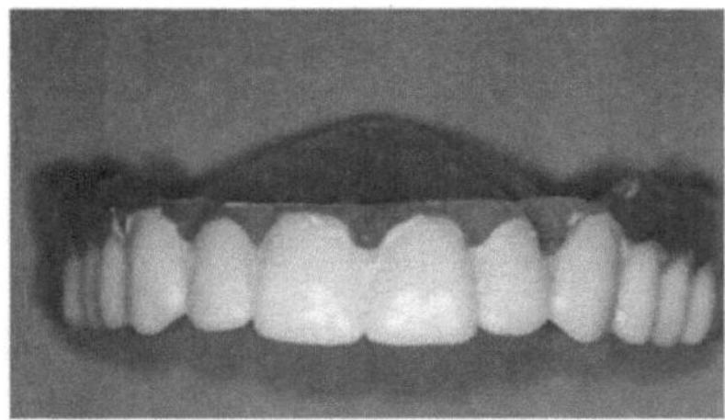

Figure 36: Anterior edge of denture removed for labial support analysis (42).

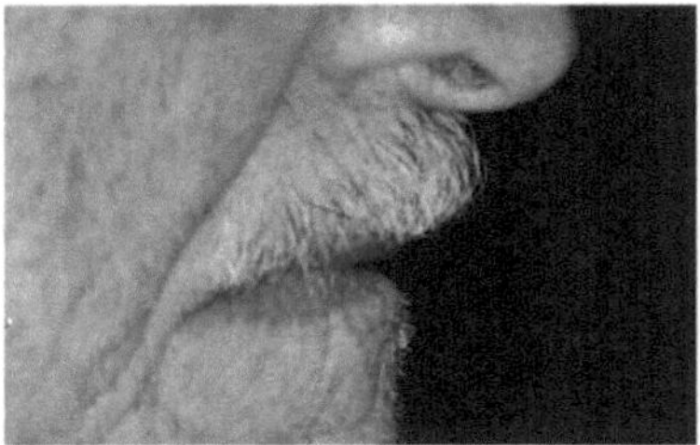

Figure 37: Side view with the duplicate in the mouth: labial support is provided by the teeth only. (42)

This method provides an effective way of visualising the level of the "gum" in relation to the neck of the future prosthetic teeth, the influence of the transition line on aesthetics, visualising lip support and getting an idea of the overall appearance of the smile and the aesthetic appearance of the future prosthesis. (42)

3-6-Prosthetic and implant planning

During the planning phase of implant surgery, the type of final restoration, the design of the prosthesis and the availability of bone and bone tissue dictate the ideal location, number, size and distribution of implants(47).Because of the absence of dental and occlusal landmarks in the edentulous patient and the resorption of the edentulous ridge, we find ourselves in a situation where no reference can give us information on the orientation and position of the implants, hence the need to use radiological and surgical guides based on the prosthetic plan. The planning of the surgical phase of implant placement is defined by the choice of implant site, the position and the ideal axes of the implants. It must be A "prosthetic-conscious" approach: the location of the implants is dictated by the prosthetic requirements of the prosthesis. Radiological and surgical guides are essential tools for successful implant placement(35).

❖ **Radiological study and radiological guide :**

Imaging is used at various stages of the implant procedure, before and after the operation, as well as during the operation itself. Imaging is an essential diagnostic element in any treatment. Various types of radiological examination are available and may be complementary. (14) Conventional imaging provides a first-line approach to the implant site: panoramic X-rays can highlight the various pathologies by visualising the entire dento-maxillary mass and can be used to assess the residual bone height in the maxilla. Profile teleradiography provides information on the offset of the bone bases or on the patient's hypo/hyper-divergent profile. (40) (14) Numerous anatomical structures of the maxilla and mandible affect and limit treatment planning and the choice of prosthesis: the height of bone available between the alveolar crest and the "critical" structure must be respected: the floor of the nasal cavities, the floor of the sinuses, the incisive foramen and canal, the mandibular canal and the chin emergence... (14) (2) In addition, thanks to planning tools, CBCT makes it possible to determine the number and size of implants and facilitates the surgical stage of implant placement thanks to surgical guides(40).The American Academy of Oral and Maxillofacial Radiology recommends cross-sectional imaging for planning implant-supported rehabilitation: CBCT is the preferred imaging method. In addition, a panoramic radiograph is recommended for the initial assessment. (40) To guarantee good results aesthetic results and functional results, implant placement planning is based on a well-conducted radiological study that includes assessment of the adjacent anatomy, and three-dimensional measurements of edentulous sites(3) This radiological study is optimised by the use of a radiological guide derived from the transparent resin duplication of a complete removable prosthesis that has been properly fitted and integrated into the edentulous crest. This guide is worn by the patient during radiological acquisition, thus improving the imaging protocol: this is the only way to match the prosthetic project with the residual bone volume: CBCT enables these implant axes to be superimposed on the bone volume. Ideally, the quantity and inclination of the bone volume should match these axes. If this is not the case, the practitioner may have to modify the axes and the choice of implant diameter and length. Planning therefore involves making a compromise between the axis of the future implants and the available bone volume. Several techniques were used in the design and manufacture of this guide. The simplest method involves making a duplicate of the patient's provisional prosthesis in transparent resin, which is used as a radiological guide. Drill holes are made along the tooth axes and parallel to each other, and filled with radiopaque material. These radiopaque markers show the axis or profile of the teeth to be replaced. (fig.38)

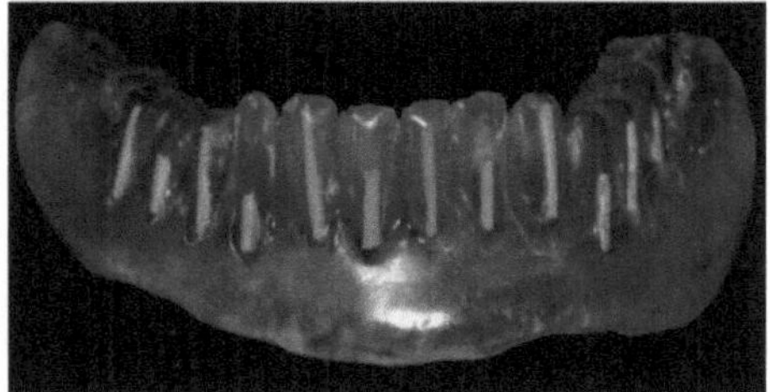

Figure 38: A clear resin duplicate of a mandibular prosthesis with radiopaque markers (gutta percha) (47)

❖ **Surgical planning: a surgical guide**

Traditional method: The radiological guide is transformed into a surgical guide: the grinding of the resin zones will allow access for the various drilling instruments and the detachment of the soft tissues (35).
Numerical method: (35) (17) (46) (65) (64)

Thanks to digital technologies, clinicians can design and manufacture surgical guides for implant placement using the "DUAL SCAN" technique. Guided surgery using these digital surgical guides requires reverse planning: starting with a total removable prosthesis defining the ideal prosthetic project, a transparent resin duplicate (radiological guide) is made and indexed by small blocks of radio-opaque material (gutta-percha) to allow digital repositioning (fig.39).

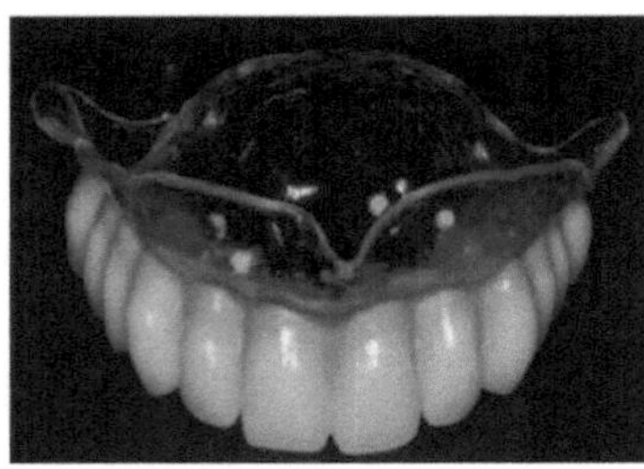

Figure 39: Indexing of the prosthetic design for the NobelGuide® system using small gutta blocks. This radiological guide enables the design to be superimposed on the bone volume by computer (35).

Surgical guides produced using the double scan method are based on two sets of data acquired in DICOM (Digital Imaging and Communication in Medicine) format. The first DICOM file comes from the patient's CBCT with the radiological guide (or prosthesis) inserted in the mouth. This radiological examination provides the bone anatomy. The second DICOM file from the CBCT of the guide alone in order to visualise the soft tissue anatomy and the position of the future teeth. This data will be used to feed the implant simulation software (Simplant, Nobel Guide, EasyGuide) and will be combined in order to choose the most ideal implant positioning and then design the surgical guide **(fig. 40 and 41)** . The adaptation and stability of the future surgical guide depends on that of the prosthesis used during the CBCT.

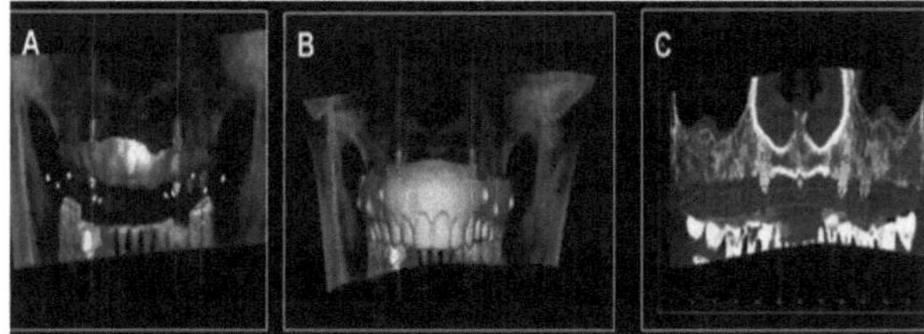

Figure 40: (A) The radiological guide/prosthesis is scanned using the "double scan" protocol, which consists of obtaining a first CBCT of the radiological guide with radiopaque markers and a second CBCT of the patient wearing the same prosthesis. (B) The two CBCT scans are then combined in the implant planning software to plan implant location and create a surgical guide. (C) Panoramic view of the planned implant sites(17)

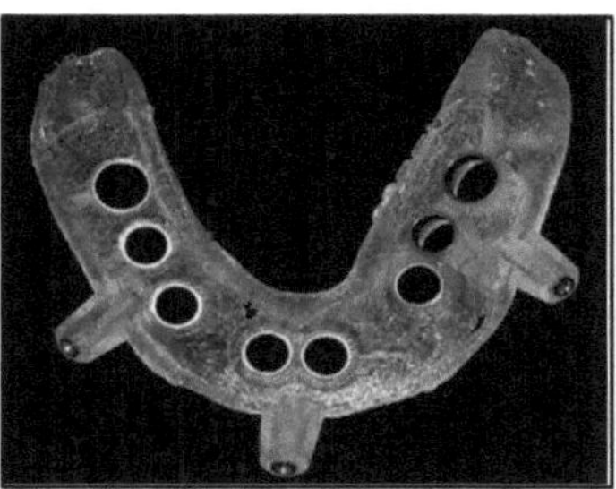

Figure 41: Radiological guide developed using the DUAL SCAN technique (Nobel Guide)(46)

The guide is stabilised in the mouth using wedges or transosseous screws. Drilling is carried out through directional cylinders of progressive diameter until the implants are in place.

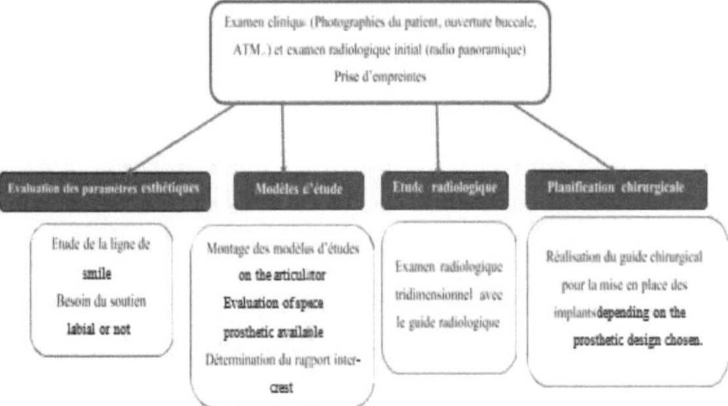

Figure 42: Preoperative assessment of supra-implant rehabilitation of the edentulous patient

CONCLUSION

Today, the supra-implant complete prosthesis is considered to be a therapy with a very good prognosis and high survival rates in the scientific literature. It is presented as a This is the preferred option for treating patients who are totally edentulous. The prosthodontist must be familiar with the various supra-implant therapeutic options in order to offer the most suitable rehabilitation to the patient, while satisfying him or her both functionally and aesthetically. Regardless of the type of prosthesis chosen, validation of a set of steps is essential to ensure the success of the total supra-implant prosthesis:

• The pre-operative stage: Clinical situations must be studied on a case-by-case basis in order to guarantee the most appropriate therapeutic solution for each patient by finding a compromise between the patient's wishes, the practitioner's skills, the prosthetic and technical possibilities and the anatomical constraints.

• The surgical phase, which includes implant placement and pre-prosthetic surgery. The planning of this phase must be "prosthetic-conscious" because it is the type of prosthesis that dictates the choice of the number and distribution of implants.

• The prosthetic stage, which consists of the design and production of the supra-implant prosthesis in line with the number and position of the implants placed, and involves close collaboration between the practitioner and the prosthetist.

Careful planning and respect for the chronology of all the stages of prosthetic-implant treatment are the keys to success. Thanks to digital workflow and the development of technologies such as CAD/CAM, the creation of a supra-implant prosthesis has become easier and more predictable: implants are placed using guided surgery, data is processed using implant planning software, virtual design and high-precision prosthetic components are manufactured. With this technology, we can save time, ensure lasting results and improve the quality of treatments.

REFERENCES

1. Abdelkoui A, Berrada S, Fajri L, Abdedine A, Merzouk N. Locator ® attachment: step-by-step clinical use in implant-stabilized removable complete prosthesis. Actual Odonto-Stomatol 2016;(280):5.

2. Alhossan A, Chang YC, Wang TJ, Wang YB, Fiorellini JP. Reliability of cone beam computed tomography in predicting implanttreatment outcomes in edentulous patients. Diagnostics 2023;13(17):2843.

3. Anadioti E, Kohltfarber H. Radiographic evaluation of prosthodontic patients.Dent Clin North Am 2021;65(3):605-21.

4. Avrampou M, Mericske-Stern R, Blatz MB, Katsoulis J.Virtual implant planning in the edentulous maxilla: criteria for decisionmaking of prosthesis design. Clin Oral Implants Res 2013;24(A100):152-9.
5. Bedrossian E, Sullivan RM, Fortin Y, Malo P, Indresano T. Fixed-prosthetic implant restoration of the edentulous maxilla: asystematic pretreatment evaluation method. J Oral Maxillofacial Surg 2008;66(1):112-22.

6. Benejam C. Supra-implant prosthesis: connectors, implant abutments and impressions. Pedagogical integration in Moodle LMS (Learning Management System). Nice: Faculté de chirurgie dentaire de Nice, 2019.

7. Bennasar B, Mahoux H, Margerit J. Complete fixed rehabilitation. Cah Prothèse 2010;150.
8. Bidra AS. Three-dimensional esthetic analysis in treatment planning for implant-supported fixed prosthesis in the edentulous maxilla: review of the esthetics literature: Three-dimensional esthetic analysis. J Esthet Restorative Dent 2011;23(4):219-36.
9. Bidra AS, Agar JR. A classification system of patients for esthetic fixed implant-supportedprostheses in the edentulous maxilla. Compend Contin Educ Dent 2010;31(5):366-8

10. Burns DR. The mandibular complete overdenture. Dent Clin North Am 2004;48(3):603-23.

11. Buser D, Sennerby L, De Bruyn H. Modern implant dentistry based on osseointegration: 50 years ofprogress, current trends and open questions. Periodontology 2000 2017;73(1):7-21.

12. Carayon D, Renaud M, Bousquet P, Montal S. Indications for supraimplant

aumaxillary complete removable prosthesis. Cah Prothèse 2015;171:37- 44.

13. Carlsson GE. Implant and root supported overdentures - a literature review and somedata on bone loss in edentulous jaws. J Adv Prosthodont 2014;6(4):245.

14. Cavézian R, Pasquet G. Cone Beam imaging and implants. Rev Stomatol Chirurgie Maxillo-faciale 2012;113(4):245-58.

15. Charrier M, De Valbray R. Stabilized supra-implant prosthesis: criteria for choosing attachment systems. Le fil dentaire 2011.

16. Davarpanah M, Martinez H. Implant options in the totally edentulous patient: criteria for choice. Implant Chir Proth 2002;8(1):79-89.

17. Deeb GR, Tran DQ, Deeb JG. Computer-Aided Planning and Placement in Implant Surgery. Atlas Oral Maxillofac Surg Clin North Am 2020;28(2):53-8.

18. Dodds M, Laborde G, Devictor A, Maille G, Sette A, MargossianP. Esthetic references: relevance from diagnosis to treatment. Prosthetic Strategy 2014;14:157-64.

19. Dudley J. Implants for the ageing population. Aust Dent J 2015;60(1):28-43.

20. Emami E, Michaud P, Sallaleh I, Feine JS. Implant-assisted complete prostheses. Periodontology 2000 2014;66(1):119-31.

21. Fajri L, Benfdil F, El Mohtarim B, El Wady W, Abdedine A. La prothèse complètemandibulaire :stabilité et rétention. Actual Odonto-Stomatol 2009;(247):267-86.

22. Felton DA. Complete edentulism and comorbid diseases: an update. J Prosthodont 2016;25(1):5-20.

23. Gray D, Patel J. Implant-supported overdentures: part 1. Br Dent J 2021;231(2):94-100.

24. Hakkoum MA, Wazir G. Telescopic dentition. Todent J 2018;12(1):246-54.

25. Haute Aotorité de la Santé. Implant-prosthetic management of edentulism: - implant-retained full-arch prosthesis - supraimplant single-unit fixed prosthesis. Saint-Denis: HAS, 2022.

26. Heckmann SM, Schrott A, Graef F, Wichmann MG, Weber H. Mandibular two-implant telescopic overdentures: 10-year clinical and radiographical results. Clin Oral Implants Res 2004;15(5):560-9.

27. Heydecke G, Zwahlen M, Nicol A et al. What is the optimal number of

implants for fixed reconstructions: asystematic review. Clin Oral Implants Res 2012;23(6):217-28.

28. Kern J, Kern T, Wolfart S, Heussen N. A systematic review and meta-analysis of removable and fixed implant-supported prostheses in edentulous jaws: post-loading implantloss. Clin Oral Implants Res 2016;27(2):174-95.

29. Kourtis S, Madianos P, Patras M, Andrikopoulou E. Rehabilitation of the edentulous mandible with implant-supported overdentures on telescopic abutments and immediate loading. A controlled prospective clinical study. J Esthet Restor Dent 2018;30(4):369-77.

30. Lago L, Rilo B, Fernández-Formoso N, DaSilva L. Implant rehabilitation planning protocol for the edentulous patientaccording to denture space, lip support, and smile line. J Prosthodontics 2017;26(6):545-8.

31. Lamy M. The edentulous maxilla. Selection criteria of an implant-supportedprosthetic rehabilitation. Rev Odonto-Stomatol 2011;40:89-101.

32. Lejeune M. Occlusal concepts in maxillary implant-supported complete prosthesis. Bordeaux: Bordeaux College of Health Sciences, 2014.

33. Leles CR, Ferreira NP, Vieira AH, Campos ACV, Silva ET. Factors influencing edentulous patients' preferences for prosthodontictreatment: Factors influencing edentulous patients' preferences. J Oral Rehabil 2011;38(5):333-9.

34. Marcelat R. The contribution of CAD/CAM in screw-retained implant prosthesis. A case study of a maxillary full bridge. Le fil dentaire 2013;(87):14-21.

35. Margossian P, Mariani P, Laborde G. Radiological and surgical guides in implantology. EMC-Odontologie 2009:1-6 [Article 23-330-A-05]
36. Martinez-Lage-Azorin Jf, Segura-Andres G, Faus Lopez J,Agustin-Panadero R. Rehabilitation with implant-supported overdentures in total edentulouspatients: a review. J Clin Exp Dent 2013;e267-72.

37. Mericske-Stern R. Prosthetic considerations.Aust Dent J 2008;53(s1).
38. Mericske-Stern R, Taylor TD, Belser U. Management of the edentulous patient. Clin Oral Implants Res 2000;11(1):108-25.

39. Millet C, Fournier J. Extracting teeth. Implant-retained complete removable prosthesis. In: Postaire M, Pompignoli M, eds. Les dernières dents : Garder ouextraire. Paris: Espace Id, 2011. p. 137-47.

40. Minassian H, Mossot L. Complete maxillary rehabilitation in implantology: the value of a checklist. Clinic 2022;43(414):1-10.

41. Morcos SS, Patel PK. The vocabulary of dentofacial deformities.Clin Plast Surg 2007;34(3):589-99.

42. Neves FD, Mendonça G, Fernandes Neto AJ. Analysis of influence of lip line and lip support in esthetics andselection of maxillary implant- supported prosthesis design. J Prosthet Dent 2004;91(3):286-8.

43. Noharet R, Clement M. Treatment of the edentulous maxilla with implant-supported fixed prosthesiswithout graft: Surgical and prosthetic aspects. Prosthetic Strategy 2014;(4):249-58.

44. N'Dindin AC, Lescher J, Bitty M, Morenas M. Total supra-implant prosthesis. Odonto-Stomatologie Tropicale 1999;85:37-43.

45. Ohkubo C, Baek KW. Does the presence of antagonist remaining teeth affect implantoverdenture success? A systematic review. J Oral Rehabil 2010;37(4):306-12.

46. Orentlicher G, Abboud M. Guided Surgery for Implant Therapy. Oral Maxillofac Surg Clin North Am 2011;23(2):239-56.

47. Patel J, Gray D. Implant-supported overdentures: part 2. Br Dent J 2021;231(3):169-75.

48. Perrin J, Sui J, Plard H, Bedouin Y, Gastard Y, Clipet F. Critères de choix pour la conception d'une suprastructure implantairede prothè se complète transvisseé. Cah Prothèse 2016;(172).

49. Richard O. Aspects biomécaniques de la prothèse implantaire fixe . Nancy: Faculté de chirurgie dentaire de Nancy, 2002.

50. Rojas-Vizcaya F. Rehabilitation of the maxillary arch with implant-supported fixed restorations guided by the most apical buccal bone level in the estheticzone: A clinical report. J Prosthet Dent 2012;107(4):213-20.

51. Rosenbaum N. Full-arch implant-retained prosthetics in general dental practice.
Dent Update 2012;39(2):108-16.

52. Sanna A, Nuytens P, Naert I, Quirynen M. Successful outcome of splinted implants supporting a 'planned' maxillary overdenture: a retrospective evaluation and comparison withfixed full dental prostheses. Clin Oral Implants Res 2009;20(4):406-13.

53. Savabi O, Nejatidanesh F, Yordshahian F. Retention of implant-supported overdenture with bar/clip and studattachment designs. J Oral Implantol

2013;39(2):140-7.

54. Scherer MD, McGlumphy EA, Seghi RR, Campagni WV.Comparison of retention and stability of two implant-retainedoverdentures based on implant location. J Prosthet Dent 2014;112(3):515-21.

55. Schwarz F, Sanz-Martín I, Kern J et al. Loading protocols and implant supported restorations proposed for the rehabilitation of partially and fully edentulous jaws. Camlog Foundation Consensus Report. Clin Oral Implants Res 2016;27(8):988-92.

56. Sikkou K, Abdelkoui A, Merzouk N, Berrada S. Preventing bone resorption for better integration of complete removable prosthetic rehabilitations. Actual Odonto-Stomatol 2016;(280):2.

57. Stiti L. Loss of retention of axial attachments in mandibular removable complete prosthesis retained by two implants: a review of the literature from 2006 to 2016. Paris Diderot : Paris faculty of dental surgery, 2017.

58. Thomason JM, Feine J, Exley C et al. Mandibular two implant-supported overdentures as the first choicestandard of care for edentulous patients - the York Consensus Statement. Br Dent J 2009;207(4):185-6.

59. Thomason JM, Kelly SAM, Bendkowski A, Ellis JS. Two implant retained overdentures--A review of the literatures supporting the McGill and York consensus statements. J Dent 2012;40(1):22-34.

60. Toquet T, Briot M. The mandibular completeupra-implant adjunctive prosthesis: current data and protocol.
Le fil dentaire 2009;(44):26-30.

61. Toquet T, Briot M, Exbrayat P. Mandibular supra-implant full denture: current data and realization protocol. Le fil dentaire 2010.

62. Tunkiwala A, Kher U, Vaidya NH. "ABCD" Implant classification: A comprehensive philosophy fortreatment planning in completely edentulous arches. J Oral Implantol 2020;46(2):93-9.

63. Turkyilmaz I, Company AM, McGlumphy EA. Should edentulous patients be constrained to removable complete dentures? The use of dental implants to improve the quality of life of edentulous patients. Gerodontology 2010;27(1):3-10.

INTERNET REFERENCES

64. Dentsplysirona. Dual Scan guidelines for taking a dental scan for SIMPLANT® [Online]. Available from URL: https://www.dentsplysirona.com/content/dam/dentsply/web/Implants/F ranchise%20Content/1222542-Dual-Scan-guidelines-for-taking-a- dental-scan-for- SIMPLANT-13vwxnb-en-1406.pdf

65. Edentulous Protocol - Dual Scan Method Scan Center. The Dual Scan method uses scan data from a patient's denture to fabricate a drill guide and is appropriate for edentulous cases where the prosthetic goal is an implant supported fixed prosthesis or hybrid [Online]. Available from URL: https://www.guidedsurgerysolutions.com/wp- content/uploads/2016/09/4b-Scan-Center-Edentulous-Dual-Scan.pdf

66. Edison Medical US. Ball Attachment Overdenture [Online]. Available from URL: https://edisonmed.com/removable- denture/ball-attachment- overdenture

67. Laboratoire Dental. Implant dentaire, implantologie [On line]. Available from URL: https://www.laboratoire- dental7.com/implantologie.php

68. NOBEL BIOCARE. Restorative concepts for edentulous patients guidelines and pre-treatment considerations for improved quality of life [Online]. Available from URL: https://www.practisdental.com/wp-content/uploads/2013/12/bedrossian-zygoma-pdf-nobel.pdf

69. Société Chirurgiens-Dentistes Sommeville. Contact the Société Chirurgiens-Dentistes Sommeville in Combs la Ville [On line]. Available from the URL: https://www.selarl- sommeville.chirurgiens-dentistes.fr/contact/

70. #maxillofacialeducation. Types of bones: maxilla and mandible [Online]. Available from URL: https://www.facebook.com/209152689630483/photos/a.251246128754 472/840002786545467/

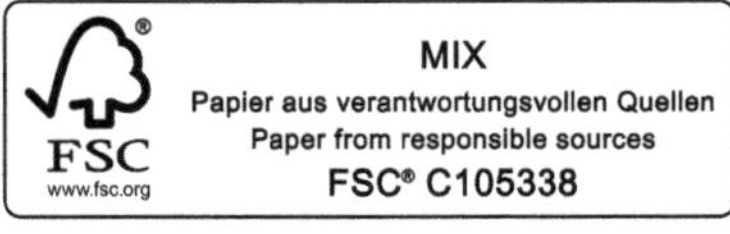

Printed by Books on Demand GmbH, Norderstedt / Germany